The Blood Sugar Solution: Blood Sugar Mastery for Long-Term Well-Being"

by

Vanessa S. Castaneda

Table of contents

Introduction

Unlocking Your Path to Blood Sugar Mastery
Welcome to a life-changing quest to manage your blood sugar and regain control of your health! This book is more than just a guide; it's your companion as you navigate the complex world of diabetes management and blood sugar control.

Understanding and regulating your blood sugar levels is a critical step towards comprehensive well-being in today's world. Whether you are dealing with diabetes or seeking preventive measures, this book is intended to provide you with knowledge, practical techniques, and a road map to long-term health.

What Makes This Book Unique:

- **Comprehensive Insights**: We delve into the complexities of blood sugar management, uncovering the science behind glucose metabolism, insulin dynamics, and the impact of lifestyle decisions on blood sugar levels. Knowledge is power, and we will provide you with the information you need to make informed health decisions.

- **Practical Guidance**: This isn't another theoretical discussion. We offer realistic, effective advice on meal planning, physical activity, and stress management, among other topics. You'll find advice and tactics that fit effortlessly into your daily life, allowing you to confidently take care of your health.
- **Personalized Approach**: We recognize that each individual is unique and will walk you through a personalized blood sugar management plan. Customize the techniques to your tastes, lifestyle, and health goals to completely personalize this trip.
- **Overall Wellness**: In addition to blood sugar control, we believe in overall wellness. You will learn how balanced eating, mindful activity, stress resilience, and proper sleep all contribute to a happy and healthy existence.

What to expect

- **Empowering Education**: Know the "why" behind each guideline so that you can make decisions that are in line with your body's demands.
- **Delectable and Packed with Nutrients**: Indulge in a variety of meals created to entice your palate while abiding by blood sugar-friendly guidelines. Taste should never be sacrificed in the name of health!
- **Interactive Tools**: Locate instruments, guides, and progress monitors that will aid you along the way. Equip yourself with tools that help you translate knowledge into practical actions.

Remember that your health is a lifelong journey, and this book is your reliable guide. Here's to uncovering the keys to stable blood sugar, embracing energy, and walking into a future where your well-being is prioritized. Let's go on this empowering journey together.

Chapter 1

An Extensive Guide to Blood Sugar Level Understanding

The fundamentals of blood sugar:

The body's main energy source is blood sugar, sometimes known as glucose. Hormones such as insulin and glucagon play a precise role in the regulation of blood sugar levels.

- **Glucose as Fuel**: Glucose from food is carried through the bloodstream to cells, providing the energy required for daily tasks.
- **Insulin's Role**: The pancreas produces insulin, which aids in the absorption of glucose into cells. This helps to reduce blood sugar levels after a meal.
- **Glucagon's Function**: The pancreas releases glucagon in response to low blood sugar, which tells the liver to

release stored glycogen as glucose. This elevates blood sugar levels.

The Value of Preserving Balance

Maintaining a precise balance of blood sugar levels is essential for overall health and well-being.

- **Energy Stability**: Maintaining healthy blood sugar levels ensures a stable and regular source of energy for body processes and activities.
- **Brain Function**: The brain is significantly reliant on glucose for energy. Stable blood sugar levels promote healthy cognitive function, concentration, and memory.
- **Complication Prevention**: Consistently high blood sugar (hyperglycemia) can cause cardiovascular illness, kidney problems, nerve damage, and vision problems, particularly in people with diabetes.
- **Hormonal Harmony**: Maintaining balanced blood sugar levels helps to

maintain hormonal balance, which guards against disruptions that can cause chronic illnesses and metabolic problems.

Effect on Overall Health:

Blood sugar levels have a significant effect on several different facets of your overall well-being.

- **Weight control**: Maintaining balanced blood sugar levels helps with weight control by decreasing the likelihood of overeating and unhealthy snacking.
- **Mood Stability**: Changes in blood sugar levels might affect mood. Maintaining balance helps to stabilize mood, which reduces the likelihood of anger and mood fluctuations.
- **Prevention of Hypoglycemia**: Low blood sugar (hypoglycemia) can cause symptoms such as shakiness and confusion. Maintaining balance helps to mitigate these detrimental impacts.

- **Increased Insulin Sensitivity**: Maintaining a balanced lifestyle that includes frequent exercise and nutritious food helps to increase insulin sensitivity, which is important for preventing type 2 diabetes and insulin resistance.
- **Optimal Physical Performance**: Balanced blood sugar levels help athletes perform at their best by ensuring that their body uses energy efficiently when they are exercising.
- **Maintenance of Overall Health**: Maintaining blood sugar within normal limits lowers the risk of chronic illnesses and increases life expectancy. It is a key component of preventive healthcare.

Chapter 2

Key Dietary Decisions for Blood Sugar Control: Healthful Eating

Blood sugar control through dietary decisions is crucial for individuals with Type 2 diabetes or who want to avoid blood sugar abnormalities. Here are some dietary guidelines to help you maintain stable blood sugar levels:

Balanced Meals: Strive for well-balanced meals, containing a mix of fats, proteins, and carbs.

- Why it matters: This well-rounded strategy can support the maintenance of steady blood sugar levels.

Complex Carbohydrate: Choose whole grains such as brown rice, quinoa, oats, and whole wheat bread over refined grains.

- Why it matters: These complex carbs promote a longer, more prolonged release of glucose, which helps to prevent sudden blood sugar increases.

Portion Control: To avoid overloading the body with carbohydrates, keep portion proportions in check.

- Why it matters: A balanced carbohydrate, protein, and fat intake can help with blood sugar regulation.

Monitor Carbohydrate: keep note of your intake and aim for consistent quantities at each meal.

- Why It Matters: Monitoring carbohydrates allows you to better regulate your blood sugar levels.

Fiber-rich Foods: Consume a range of foods high in fiber, such as whole grains, fruits, vegetables, and legumes, throughout your diet.

- Why it matters: Carbohydrate digestion and absorption are slowed down by fiber, which helps to stabilize blood sugar levels.

Lean Proteins: Choose lean protein sources such as fish, chicken, tofu, lentils, and low-fat dairy.

- Why it matters: Protein slows down the breakdown and absorption of carbohydrates, which helps to stabilize blood sugar levels.

Nutritious Fats: Include foods high in unsaturated fats, like olive oil, nuts, seeds, and avocados.

- Why it matters: Nutritious fats aid in regulating appetite and bring balance to the diet.

Consistent Meal Timing: Maintain a regular meal plan with meals spaced out equally throughout the day.

- Why it matters: This gives the body a constant supply of nutrients, which helps control blood sugar levels.

Minimize added Sugars: Reduce your intake of sugary foods and beverages. Choose natural sweeteners like honey or maple syrup in moderation, and be wary of hidden sugars in processed meals.

- Why it matters: Excess sugar can cause blood sugar to rise and have a detrimental influence on general health.

Smart Snacking: Select high-nutrient snacks such as fresh veggies, Greek yogurt, or almonds.

- Why It Matters: Eating a nutritious snack can help reduce blood sugar swings during the day.

Staying Hydrated: Consume a lot of water to stay hydrated because dehydration might lower blood sugar levels. Water, herbal teas, or other low-calorie liquids are preferable to sugary drinks.

- Why it matters: Proper hydration promotes general health and improves blood circulation.

Low-Glycemic Index Foods: Choose foods that have a lower glycemic index since they have less of an effect on blood sugar levels. Sweet potatoes and other non-starchy veggies are some of the examples.

- Why it matters: This causes a slower, more gradual increase in blood sugar levels, improving overall blood sugar control.

Test and Learn: Regularly check blood sugar levels to learn individual reactions to foods.

- Why it Matters: Testing allows you to fine-tune your meal plan for maximum blood sugar control.

Meal planning: Plan your meals ahead of time to guarantee a healthy and balanced diet. This helps prevent impulsive, unhealthy meal decisions.

Chapter 3

Physical Activity and Blood Sugar: Exercise for Level Management

Regular physical activity is an effective technique for regulating blood sugar levels, particularly for individuals with diabetes or those seeking to avoid blood sugar imbalances. Here's how exercise helps and how to include physical activity in your daily routine:

Exercise's Function in Blood Sugar Regulation:

- Enhanced Insulin Sensitivity: As a result of regular exercise, cells are better able to utilize glucose, and blood sugar regulation is enhanced.
- Muscle Glucose Uptake: Exercise encourages the muscles to absorb glucose, which lowers blood sugar levels. After exercise, this impact may persist for several hours.

- Weight control: Exercise helps people lose or maintain their weight, which is important for avoiding insulin resistance and type 2 diabetes, which are conditions linked to obesity.
- Improved Blood Circulation: Improved blood circulation promotes the effective delivery of glucose to cells, hence improving glucose homeostasis.
- Increased Glucagon Action: Exercise enhances the action of glucagon, a hormone that elevates blood sugar levels, which helps to maintain glucose management balance.

Tips for Including Physical Activity:

Select activities you enjoy:

- Why It Matters: Choose exercises that you enjoy to improve your commitment to your plan.
- Suggestions: Try walking, running, cycling, swimming, or group classes.

Begin gradually.

- Why It Matters: Beginning with low-impact activities and gradually increasing intensity can prevent injury and increase endurance over time.
- Suggestions: Start with simple activities like brisk walking or easy yoga before advancing to more intense exercises.

Set realistic goals:

- Why it Matters: Establishing achievable goals helps encourage and track progress.
- Suggestions: Set precise goals, such as getting a certain number of minutes of exercise every day or reaching certain milestones.

Incorporate Variety:

- Why It Matters: Combine aerobic exercises (e.g., walking or biking) with strength training for overall health benefits.

- Suggestions: Change up your program by combining aerobic and resistance activities.

Be constant:

- Why It Matters: Exercise that is constant and regular is essential for long-lasting reductions in blood sugar levels.
- Suggestions: Try to get in at least 150 minutes a week, spaced out across multiple days, of moderate-intensity activity.

Check blood sugar levels:

- Why It Matters: Consistent monitoring facilitates understanding of the effects of various exercises on blood sugar levels and enables necessary modifications.
- Suggestions: If you have diabetes in particular, check your blood sugar levels both before and after working out.

Examine Timing:

- Why It Matters: Exercise's effect on blood sugar levels can be influenced by when it is done.
- Suggestions: Try varying the times of day to observe when your body reacts most favorably.

Stay Hydrated:

- Why It Matters: Proper hydration promotes general health and improves blood circulation during activity.
- Suggestion: Drink water before, during, and after exercise.

Consultation for Diabetes Management:

- Why It Matters: For individualized exercise regimens, people with diabetes should speak with healthcare providers.
- Suggestions: Customize your exercise regimen in consultation with a licensed fitness professional or your healthcare physician.

Chapter 4

Sugar and Sweeteners: Knowledge of Effects on Blood Sugar Levels and Better Substitutes

The Effects of Various Sugars on Blood Sugar Levels:

- Sucrose (table sugar): Consisting of glucose and fructose, sucrose rapidly boosts blood sugar levels when ingested. Individuals with diabetes should keep their sugar intake minimal.

- High-Fructose Corn Syrup (HFCS): HFCS is frequently found in processed foods and sugary beverages. It has been linked to insulin resistance and an increased risk of metabolic complications.

- Fructose: While naturally occurring in fruits, excessive fructose consumption may contribute to insulin resistance and high blood triglyceride levels. The impact, however, may alter when ingested in whole fruits due to fiber content.

- Artificial Sweeteners: Aspartame, saccharin, and sucralose are non-nutritive sweeteners that give sweetness without adding calories. They normally have little effect on blood sugar levels and can be useful choices for diabetics.

Nutritious Substitutions for Refined Sugar:

- Stevia: A natural sweetener derived from the Stevia rebaudiana plant's leaves, stevia does not affect blood sugar and can be an excellent option for people looking for a non-caloric sweetener.
- Monk Fruit: Luo Han Guo, also known as monk fruit extract, is a calorie-free natural sweetener. It does not raise blood sugar levels and can be used as a sugar replacement.
- Erythritol: A sugar alcohol with fewer calories, erythritol has no notable effect on blood sugar. It's widely used in low-calorie and sugar-free products.

- Agave Nectar: Although lower on the glycemic index than table sugar, agave nectar should be used in moderation due to its high fructose concentration.
- Maple syrup and honey: These natural sweeteners have a lower glycemic index than refined sugars, but should be used in moderation. They also include more nutrients than processed sugars.

Considerations for Diabetes Patients:

- Glycemic Index: Selecting foods with a lower Glycemic index can aid in better control of blood sugar levels.
- Portion Control: Moderation is key, even when using healthier substitutes. Pay attention to portion proportions to prevent consuming too many calories and carbohydrates.
- Individual Reactions: Each person's experience with sweeteners is unique. Assessing blood sugar levels regularly can assist in figuring out individual tolerances.

Engage in Professional Consultation:

- Diabetics should consult with healthcare experts or registered dietitians before making significant adjustments to their sweetener preferences. Personalized guidance can take into account specific health issues as well as individual reactions.

Chapter 5

Supplements and Herbs for Blood Sugar Control: Investigating Natural Support

Blood sugar levels must be managed carefully, and several natural vitamins and herbs may help. It is critical to contact a healthcare practitioner before adopting these into your routine, especially if you have pre-existing health conditions or are taking medication. Consider the following vitamins and herbs:

Cinnamon:

- Potential Advantages: Cinnamon may enhance insulin sensitivity, assisting cells in responding to insulin and controlling blood sugar more effectively.
- Usage: This supplement can be consumed or added to a diet. For greater health advantages, go for Ceylon cinnamon.

Berberine:

- Potential Advantages: Berberine may have an impact on blood sugar regulation by enhancing insulin sensitivity.
- Usage: Supplements are frequently offered. To find out the right dosages, speak with a medical practitioner.

Chromium:

- Potential Advantages: Chromium may improve insulin sensitivity through its role in glucose metabolism.
- Usage: It is available as a supplement. Ensure that you meet the recommended daily allowance through a combination of diet and supplementation.

Alpha-Lipoic Acid:

- Potential Advantages: Acts as an antioxidant and may enhance insulin sensitivity.

- Usage: As a supplement, it is possible to consume. For advice on the right dosages, see a medical professional.

Gymnema Sylvestre:

- Potential Advantages: Gymnema may help minimize sugar absorption in the intestines and improve insulin activity.
- Usage: Available as a supplement. Consult a healthcare practitioner for specific dosing instructions.

Bitter Melon:

- Potential Advantages m: Bitter melon has ingredients that may reduce blood sugar levels.
- Usage: As a vegetable or supplement, bitter melon can be taken as directed. Consult a healthcare professional about optimal usage.

Fenugreek:

- Potential Advantages: Fenugreek has the potential to reduce blood sugar and enhance insulin sensitivity.
- Usage: Often eaten as a supplement or as a spice. For dose information, speak with a medical practitioner.

Magnesium:

- Potential Advantages: Magnesium aids in glucose metabolism and insulin action.
- Usage: Eat a well-balanced diet with adequate amounts of magnesium, or consider taking supplements if necessary. Speak with a healthcare provider.

Aloe Vera:

- Potential Advantages: Aloe vera may reduce blood sugar levels, but additional research is needed.
- Usage: Available as a supplement. Consult a healthcare practitioner to determine the optimum dosage.

Turmeric (Curcumin):

- Prospective Advantages: The active ingredient in turmeric, curcumin, may have the ability to reduce inflammation and control blood sugar.
- Use: May be taken as a supplement or added to food. Make sure you take it with black pepper for optimal absorption.

Chapter 6

Managing Stress and Blood Sugar

Understanding the Connection

The intricate connection between stress and blood sugar levels suggests that stress may have an effect on blood glucose management in the short and long term. For improved general health, consider the following summary and stress-reduction strategies:

1. **Stress and blood sugar level;**

Cortisol Release: Stress causes the release of stress hormones, including cortisol and adrenaline. These hormones can elevate blood sugar levels by causing the liver to produce glucose.

Insulin Resistance: Chronic stress may cause cells to become less receptive to insulin. This can cause high blood sugar levels over time.

Emotional Eating: Stress can cause emotional

eating or poor food choices, affecting overall dietary habits and blood sugar regulation.

2. **Stress Management Techniques**:

Frequent Exercise:

- Advantages: Exercise lowers stress hormones and encourages endorphin release, which lifts mood.
- Suggestions: Include workouts you enjoy in your schedule, such as yoga, jogging, walking, or other physical activities.

Mindfulness and Meditation:

- Advantages: Mindfulness practices and meditation help reduce stress and foster a state of calm.
- Suggestions: Practice deep breathing techniques, guided meditation, or mindfulness activities regularly.

Relaxation Methods:

- Advantages: Techniques such as progressive muscle relaxation or deep breathing can help the body relax and reduce tension.
- Suggestions: Schedule time for relaxation activities, especially during stressful times.

Sufficient Sleep:

- Advantages: Stress reduction and general wellness depend on getting enough sleep.
- Suggestions: Aim for 7-9 hours of sleep per night, establish a regular sleep schedule, and provide a cozy sleeping space.

Social Support:

- Advantages: Reaching out to loved ones, friends, or a counselor offers psychological support and aids in stress reduction.
- Suggestions: Establish deep social ties and be honest when discussing stressors.

Good Nutrition:

- Advantages: An appropriately balanced diet not only promotes general health but also has a favorable impact on stress and mood.
- Suggestions: Consume foods high in nutrients, drink enough water, and keep away from processed foods and too much caffeine.

Time Management:

- Advantages: Effective time management decreases stress from deadlines and pressures.
- Suggestions: Prioritize things, break them down into smaller parts, and make achievable targets.

Hobbies and Leisure Activities:

- Advantages: Indulging in pleasurable pursuits offers a means of relieving stress.
- Suggestions: Schedule a regular time for interests or pastimes you enjoy.

Counseling and Therapy:

- Advantages: Expert assistance can assist people in learning coping mechanisms and managing stress.
- Suggestions: If necessary, think about obtaining counseling or treatment.

3. Consistency is Important:

Use stress management techniques consistently for long-term results.

Tailor techniques to your interests and lifestyle, and find out what works best for you.

Chapter 7

Handling Blood Sugar at Home: A Comprehensive Guide to Accurate Self-Testing

Individuals with diabetes and those at risk of blood sugar imbalances should monitor their blood sugar levels at home regularly. Here's a detailed guide on how to accurately check blood sugar at home:

Regular testing is important;

- Early Discovery: Regular monitoring enables the early discovery of variations in blood sugar levels, allowing for timely adjustments to treatment regimens or lifestyles.
- Treatment Adjustments: Understanding blood sugar patterns enables healthcare practitioners to make required changes to medications, insulin dosages, and lifestyle advice.

- Complication Prevention: Regular monitoring helps to avoid consequences associated with high or low blood sugar, such as cardiovascular disease, kidney damage, and nerve disorders.
- Personal Empowerment: Home monitoring enables people to actively participate in their diabetes management, which leads to a greater awareness of how lifestyle choices affect blood sugar levels.

Choosing a Glucometer;

- Accuracy: Select a glucometer that has a history of accuracy. Verify that it satisfies industry requirements and has undergone the correct calibration.
- Ease of Use: Choose a gadget that is simple to use, has easy handling instructions, and is easy to understand.
- Testing Strips Compatibility: Verify that the glucometer's testing strips are affordable and easily accessible.
- Data Storage: A few glucometers have memory functions that allow you to save

prior readings and monitor trends over time.

When and How Often to Test;

- Fasting blood sugar: usually checked first thing in the morning, before a meal or drink.
- Postprandial Blood Sugar: Checked two hours following a meal to see how the body handles carbohydrates.
- Before and After Exercise: It's crucial for those who are managing their diabetes to know how exercise affects blood sugar levels.
- As directed by the healthcare provider: adhere to the testing regimen your healthcare provider suggests, taking into account your specific medical requirements.

Proper Blood Sampling Method;

- Wash your hands: To prevent contamination, make sure your hands are clean and dry before testing.
- Lance the Side of the Fingertip: Prick the side of the fingertip with a lancet. Rotate your fingers to reduce pain.
- Gather a little blood sample: Apply a little droplet of blood to the testing strip after letting it develop.
- Observe the instructions on the device: For accurate readings, place the strip into the glucometer and follow the directions unique to your device.

Interpreting the Results;

- Goal levels: Follow your healthcare provider's recommendations on goal blood sugar levels.
- Patterns and Trends: Throughout time, keep an eye out for patterns and trends in your readings. Take note of how food, exercise, and other elements affect you.
- Speak with the healthcare provider: Consult your healthcare professional for

advice regarding any worries or inquiries you may have regarding your readings.

Record-keeping;

- Keep a log: Record the date, time, and any notes you make regarding your activities or meals, along with your blood sugar readings.
- Give to the Healthcare Provider: During routine check-ups, share your record with your healthcare provider so they can evaluate your diabetes management in greater detail.

Frequent Maintenance and Calibration;

- Check Expiry Dates: Make sure that testing strips and lancets are not past their expiration dates.
- Calibrate the Glucometer: To guarantee accuracy, calibrate the device regularly according to the manufacturer's recommendations.

- Device Maintenance: To guarantee correct operation, keep the glucometer clean and adhere to maintenance guidelines.

One of the most effective ways to manage diabetes and advance general health is to regularly check your blood sugar at home. Individuals can make well-informed judgments regarding their treatment programs and lifestyle by actively engaging in self-monitoring.

Conclusion

Your path to a blood sugar solution
"The Blood Sugar Solution: Blood Sugar Mastery for Long-Term Well-Being" is a complete guide to help you on your journey to vibrant health. This book is your companion to long-term well-being, from understanding the science of blood sugar to implementing practical measures adapted to your lifestyle. Personalize your route, embrace a holistic lifestyle, and confidently face a future of long-term health. Your journey to the Blood Sugar Solution awaits a symphony of regulated blood sugar and eternal vitality.